I0435423

Weight Loss Secrets and Strategies: Gluten-Free Fat Burning Recipes to Lose Weight Quickly

Disclaimer and Terms of Use: Effort has been made to ensure that the information in this book is accurate and complete, however, the author and the publisher do not warrant the accuracy of the information, text and graphics contained within the book due to the rapidly changing nature of science, research, known and unknown facts and internet. The Author and the publisher do not hold any responsibility for errors, omissions or contrary interpretation of the subject matter herein. This book is presented solely for motivational and informational purposes only.

Table of Contents

Introduction

Fat burning is a process that reduces fat stores in our body. Fat burning occurs under two different circumstances.

Primarily, fats are burnt during exercise or workouts. The cells utilize the fats as a fuel for releasing energy required by the body to perform various activities. When the activities are intense, the fat burning process also becomes intense.

Fat burning also occurs during the process of digestion. In order to digest the foods, our body burns the fat to release energy. This energy is used for digestion. However, the fats that are burnt during digestion are quite less compared to the nutrients, sugar and fats obtained from the food.

On the other hand, there are certain low-calorie or fat-free foods that does not contain any fat contents. In order to digest such foods, our body might need to burn more fats. In short, consumption of such food items helps in reducing weight. Such food items are known as fat-burning foods. Fat-burning recipes are made using such food items.

Effects Of Gluten

Over the past couple of years, several studies are conducted on food items that contain gluten.

Gluten is a type of protein which is found in different types of grains. The most common grain that contains gluten is wheat. Gluten is also found in rye, barley and a hybrid grain called triticale.

Scientific studies have proved that consumption of gluten in large quantities can cause several problems. Gluten contains certain substances that kill the useful bacteria in our intestine which are known as probiotics. This leads to increase in harmful bacteria. Lack of probiotics also leads to slow digestion. It also gives rise to several other problems like constipation.

Gluten causes severe symptoms in people who suffer from celiac disease.

Some people suffer from wheat intolerance. For such people it is better to avoid foods that contain gluten.

Similarly, there is a skin disorder known as Dermatitis Herpetiformis which is characterized by red and inflamed skin. Consumption of gluten can cause serious symptoms in those who suffer from this skin disorder.

Gluten Free Fat-Burning Recipes

Fat-burning recipes are always in demand. However, with the spread of awareness about the harmful effects of gluten, people are looking for gluten-free food remedies. In this review we will be discussing about few fat-burning recipes that are gluten-free.

These recipes can help you in actively including differing types of fat-burning foods into your regular diet. However, for a faster weight loss you should follow some exercise routines along with diet control. Avoid foods that are high in fat. Also avoid fried and roasted foods that are high in calories and fat.

This is a simple breakfast recipe that you can make within 15 minutes. Broccoli used in this recipe is rich in dietary fiber and it also contains lots of antioxidants. The egg whites are rich in protein and other nutrients. This menu can leave you satisfied until afternoon.

Ingredients:

Cooking spray.

Chopped broccoli – 1 cup.

2 eggs (remove the egg yolks)

Crumbled feta – 2 tbsp.

Dried dill – ¼ tbsp.

Toasted bread.

Preparation

Heat a non-stick pan for few minutes and coat it using cooking spray. Add the chopped broccoli and cook for around 4 to 5 minutes.

Take a small bowl and make a mixture of egg whites, dill and feta. Add this mixture to the broccoli in the pan. Again cook for 4 to 5 minutes. Flip the omelet and let it stay for 2 more minutes.

Your fat-burning omelet is ready. You can have it with bread or toast.

Salmon Noodle

Ingredients

Buckwheat noodles - 4 ounces.

Chopped asparagus – 5 ounces.

Cooking spray.

Salmon fillet – 8 pieces.

Sesame oil.

Lime juice – 3 tbsp.

Kosher salt – 1/4th tbsp.

Fresh pepper – 1/4th tbsp.

Cucumber pieces – 4 ounces.

1/2 Avocado, chopped.

This recipe contains several ingredients that can help in boosting your metabolism. Avocado and salmon contains healthy fats. Vegetables and noodles contain dietary fiber. Asparagus contains vitamin A and C, minerals, iron and folate.

Preparation

Boil water in a bowl and add the noodles. Once the noodles are cooked transfer them into another bowl. Similarly, cook asparagus and keep it aside.

Heat a non-stick pan over medium heat. Coat the pan using cooking spray. Now cook the pieces of salmon and keep it aside.

Heat sesame oil along with pepper, salt and lime juice. To this mixture add asparagus and noodles. Stir it for few minutes.

Now add avocado and cucumber. Toss it for few minutes. Then add the salmon.

Your fat-burning dish is ready.

Chickpea Slaw

Chickpea slaw is very healthy and full of nutrients. You can prepare this as your lunch or for your dinner. Chickpeas contain lots of proteins and dietary fiber. This is an amazing fat-burning recipe that can keep you satisfied until evening.

Ingredients

Fat-free yogurt –1/4 cup.

Cider vinegar –1/4th tbsp.

Water – 1 tbsp.

Black pepper- freshly grounded.

Low-sodium chickpeas – 1 Can.

Sliced cabbage- 2 1/2 cups.

Celery- 2 stalks, thinly sliced.

Sliced carrots -2

Toasted sesame seeds – 2 tbsp.

Preparation

Take a bowl and add yogurt, water, pepper, salt and vinegar. Mix these items and then add chickpeas, celery, cabbage and carrots. Toss them well. Now add sesame seeds.

Your slaw is ready. But you need to refrigerate it for 4 to 5 hours before you serve it.

Grapefruit And Banana

Grapefruit aids in faster weight loss. It contains lot of water which fills you up and thus it helps you in avoiding overeating.

Ingredients

Refrigerated grapefruit sections – 2 cups.

Sliced banana – 1 cup.

Chopped mint – 1 tbsp.

Honey – 1 tbsp.

Preparation

Take few grapefruit sections and squeeze them to make 1/4th cup of juice.

Mix the juice with banana slices and remaining grapefruit sections. Add honey and mint and refrigerate for some time. Your fruit salad is ready.

Kidney Beans, Sausage And Chili

Red kidney beans and chili powder helps in burning fat. Kidney beans are also rich in proteins. Chili contains capsaicin which helps in boosting your metabolism.

Ingredients

Turkey Italian sausage- 6 ounces

Chopped onion – 2 cups.

Green bell pepper, chopped – 1 cup.

Minced garlic cloves – 8.

Ground sirloin – 1 pound.

Chopped jalapeno pepper – 1

Chili powder – 2 tbsp.

Brown sugar – 2 tbsp.

Ground cumin – 1 tbsp.

Tomato paste – 3 tbsp.

Dried oregano – 1 tbsp.

Black pepper (freshly ground) – 1/2 tbsp.

Salt – 1/4 tbsp.

Bay leaves – 2

Red wine – 1 1/4 cups.

Chopped tomatoes – 2 cups.

Drained kidney beans – 2 cups.

Shredded cheddar cheese – 1/2 cup.

Preparation

Heat an oven with medium heat. Add sausage, green bell pepper, onion, minced garlic cloves, sirloin and jalapeno pepper. Cook for around 10 minutes. Allow the sausage to turn brownish.

Add brown sugar, chili powder, cumin, tomato paste, oregano, black pepper, salt and bay leaves. Cook for couple of minutes and stir well. Then add chopped tomatoes, kidney beans and red wine and stir till the mixture begins to boil. Now cover the pan with a lid and reduce the flame. Let it cook for 1 hour.

Uncover the pan and stir the mixture. Let it cook for another 30 minutes. Remove the bay leaves and add cheddar cheese.

You can preserve it for the next day too.

White Bean Hummus

You can make healthy and nutritious hummus at your home using fat-burning foods and delicious veggies.

Ingredients

Drained white beans – 1/4 cup.

Chopped chives – 1 tbsp.

Lemon juice – 1 tbsp.

Olive oil – 2 tbsp.

Chopped baby carrots – 2

Broccoli florets – 1/2 cup.

Sliced green pepper.

Sliced red pepper.

Preparation

Mix white beans with lemon juice, chives and olive oil. Mash this mixture using a fork.

You can have this with vegetable salads made of cucumbers, sugar snap peas, carrots, broccoli, bell peppers and grape tomatoes.

Turkey Burger

Turkey is a rich source of healthy lean protein. This special turkey burger will reduce your craving for red meat. Turkey is also a source of amino acids which help in building muscles.

Ingredients

Dark-meat turkey - 1 pound.

Minced garlic clove – 1

Paprika - 1/2 tbsp.

Ground cumin - 1/4 tbsp.

Kosher salt.

Black pepper (freshly ground) – 1/4 tbsp.

Grilled sweet onion slices.

Barbecue sauce – 1/4 cup.

Sesame seed buns.

Preparation

Take a bowl and mix the turkey with paprika, garlic and cumin.

Divide the turkey into 4-inch long patties.

Season the turkey pieces using salt and pepper.

Grill the turkey pieces until they are well cooked.

Use onions, cabbage and tomatoes for toppings.

Your low-fat burger is ready.

Rice Salad

This is a simple dish that can be easily made. Chickpea is one of the main ingredients of this recipe. You can have this dish as a lunch or dinner. It is fulfilling and tasty and it doesn't contain any kind of high-calorie ingredient.

Ingredients

Olive oil – 2 tbsp.

Sliced sweet onion – 3/4 cup.

Drained chickpeas – 1 Can.

Ground cumin – 1/2 tbsp.

Salt – 1/4 tbsp.

Black pepper, freshly ground.

Brown rice (cooked) – 3 cups.

Chopped dates – 1/2 cup.

Chopped mint – 1/4 cup.

Chopped parsley – 1/4 cup.

Preparation

Heat olive oil in a non-stick pan. Add sliced onion and keep stirring until the onions turn brownish in color. Cut off the flames and add chickpeas, salt and cumin. Stir nicely and add the black pepper.

To this mixture add the cooked rice, chopped dates, parsley and mint. Toss well and serve warm.

Quinoa And Black Beans

Quinoa is a gluten-free whole grain which is rich in dietary fiber and protein. It helps in maintaining your metabolism. Similarly, black beans are also a good source of dietary fiber. This dish is spicy and delicious and it can certainly replace your high-calorie lunch or dinner.

Ingredients

Cooked quinoa – 1 cup

Rinsed and drained black beans – 1/3 cup

Chopped tomato – 1

Sliced scallion – 1

Olive oil – 1 tbsp.

Lemon juice – 1 tbsp.

Salt to taste.

Black pepper, freshly ground – 1/4 tbsp.

Preparation

Heat olive oil in a non-stick pan. Add black beans to it. Stir for few minutes. Add tomatoes, scallion, cooked quinoa, salt and black pepper. Toss well and cut the flame. Sprinkle it with lemon juice and serve hot.

Banana, Barley And Sunflower Seeds.

If you are tired of your regular breakfast menu, get ready to try something new and healthy. This special recipe made of banana and barley contains resistant starch and lots of fiber. It is definitely an ideal breakfast that can boost your metabolism.

Ingredients

Water – 2/3 cup.

Pearl barley – 1/3 cup.

Sliced banana – 1.

Sunflower seeds – 1 tbsp.

Honey – 1 tbsp.

Preparation

Add the water to the barely and cook for 10 minutes.

Drain excess water and add the slices of banana, honey and sunflower seeds to it.

Your fat-burning breakfast is ready.

Greek Yogurt And Fruit Parfait

If you are on a weight loss regimen, then it is highly beneficial to add more fruits to your regular diet. This special fruit parfait is not only a rich source of energy but it can also help you in reducing your weight. The Greek yogurt in this special recipe can fulfill your calorie requirement and keep you satisfied for 4 to 6 hours.

Ingredients

Fat-free Greek yogurt – 1 cup.

Sliced nectarines, peaches and plums – 2 cups.

Puffed rice – 3/4 cup.

Toasted and finely chopped walnuts – 1 tbsp.

Toasted and finely chopped almonds – 1 tbsp.

Ground flaxseed – 1 tbsp.

Maple Syrup – 1 tbsp.

Honey - 1 tbsp.

Preparation

Take a big jar or container and fill it with 1/2 cup of yogurt. On top of it add a layer of sliced nectarines, peaches and plums. Then add a layer of puffed rice. Follow this with nuts and flaxseeds. Finally pour half of the maple syrup.

Again start with yogurt. Add the remaining 1/2 cup of yogurt and spread it into a layer. Repeat the layers as above. You can top it with more puffed rice to make it crunchier.

Green Tea Smoothie

Green tea is popular for its weight loss benefits. It contains an active ingredient, EGCG which helps in boosting metabolism. For this reason, it is important to include green tea in your daily routine in order to achieve faster weight loss. This is a delicious smoothie which contains cayenne spices, agave nectar and lime juice.

Ingredients

Boiled green tea – 3/4 cup.

Cayenne pepper – 1/8 tbsp.

Lemon juice – 1 tbsp.

Agave nectar – 2 tbsp.

Chopped pear – 1

Fat-free yogurt – 2 tbsp.

Ice cubes – 7

Preparation

Add all the aforementioned ingredients into a blender and blend well. Your fat-burning smoothie is done.

Curried Egg Sandwich

Eggs form an important part of weight-loss diet. They are delicious and satisfying. They are rich in protein and low in calories. This special egg sandwich is a perfect replacement for your lunch. Instead of mayo we have used fat-free Greek yogurt. So, here is how it is done.

Ingredients

Cooked and chopped eggs – 2

Fat-free Greek yogurt – 2 tbsp.

Red bell pepper (chopped) – 2 tbsp.

Curry powder – 1/4 tbsp.

Salt – 1/8 tbsp.

Pepper – 1/8 tbsp.

Toasted bread – 2 slices.

Chopped spinach – 1/2 cup.

Preparation

Take a small bowl and add yogurt, eggs, bell pepper, salt, curry powder and pepper. Mix all these ingredients and stir well.

Put spinach on the bread and then place the egg salad.

Chicken Chilaquiles And Black Beans

It is a conventional Mexican breakfast. Despite all the ingredients it comes below 300 calories. Since it is baked it is totally safe for the weight conscious lot. The black beans used in this recipe contain proteins and lots of fiber. Although it is a breakfast item, you can have it for lunch or dinner.

Ingredients

Cooking spray

Sliced onion – 1 cup

Minced garlic cloves – 5.

Cooked and shredded chicken breast – 2 cups.

Drained black beans – 1 Can.

Fat-free chicken broth – 1 cup.

Salsa de chile fresco – 1 Can

Chopped corn tortillas – 15.

Queso blanco (shredded) – 1 cup.

Preparation

Heat a non-stick pan over average heat. Coat the pan using cooking spray. Add sliced onions and sauté them for 5 minutes. Next, add minced garlic and sauté for 2 minutes. Then add the shredded chicken and cook for 1 minute. Now transfer this to a bigger bowl. Add the beans and stir well. Now boil salsa and broth in a pan. Reduce the flame and cook for 5 minutes.

Put some tortilla strips on a baking dish. Now add some chicken mixture to it. Now add the rest of the chicken and tortillas. Next, pour the broth mixture. Add some cheese on the top. Now bake it at around 450 degree for about 10 minutes.

Black Bean With Tomato Soup

This special soup is made from black beans which is a great food for weight-conscious eaters. It contains lots of proteins and fiber. This recipe also contains jalapenos and chili powder.

Ingredients

Olive oil – 2 tbsp.

Chopped onion – 1 1/2 cups.

Seeded jalapeno (chopped) – 1 cup.

Chopped garlic clove – 1.

Chili powder – 1 tbsp.

Ground cumin – 1 tbsp.

Tomato soup and red pepper (roasted) – 32 ounces.

Drained black beans – 2 Cans.

Sour cream – 1/4 cup.

Chopped Cilantro – 1/4 cup.

Cilantro sprigs. 1/2 cup.

Preparation

Heat a large non-stick pan and pour the olive oil. Heat the oil for some time and then add the jalapeno and chopped onions. Cook for around 3 minutes. Add chopped garlic, cumin and chili powder. Cook for few minutes. Next, add black beans and soup. Reduce the flame and cook for 5 minutes. Next, add cilantro.

Pour the soup into a bowl and add the sour cream and cilantro sprigs.

Creamy Avocado

This is a simple recipe which is extremely low in calories. This dish is extremely filling and it would leave you satisfied for several hours.

Ingredients

Avocado – 1

Lime juice – 1 tbsp.

Plain yogurt or sour cream – 1 tbsp.

Ground cumin – 1/4 tbsp.

Chopped cilantro – 1 tbsp.

Endive leaves – 12.

Preparation

Peel the avocado and mash it to make a paste.

Take a bowl and mix lime juice sour cream, cumin and cilantro. Now add the mashed avocado and stir well.

Place this mixture into the endive leaves.

Salmon And Pineapple Salsa

Salmon is a rich source of lean protein which is important for building muscles. This is a highly nourishing diet for weight-conscious eaters. Salmon also contains monounsaturated fats. This can help in better weight reduction.

Ingredients

Chopped pineapple – 1 cup.

Red onion, finely chopped – 2 tbsp.

Chopped cilantro – 2 tbsp.

Rice vinegar – 1 tbsp.

Red pepper, ground – 1/8 tbsp.

Cooking spray.

Salmon fillets – 4.

Salt – 1/2 teaspoon.

Preparation

In a medium-size bowl add chopped pineapples, red onion, cilantro, rice vinegar and red pepper. Stir well and keep it aside.

Heat a grill pan over medium fire. Coat the pan using cooking spray. Place the fish pieces and sprinkle them with salt. Cook for 10 minutes and then top the pieces with salsa.

Garbanzo Salad

This Mediterranean salad is quite nutritious and low in calories. This salad contains low-fat dairy, fresh vegetables, lean proteins and healthy fats. A single serving of this special salad contains around 159 calories.

Ingredients

Fennel bulb, finely chopped – 3 cups

Chopped tomato – 2 cups.

Red onion, finely chopped – 1 3/4 cups.

Chopped basil – 1 cup.

Balsamic vinegar – 1/3 cup.

Olive oil – 1 tbsp.

Black pepper, freshly ground – 1 tbsp.

Salt – 1/4 tbsp.

Minced garlic – 4 cloves.

Drained garbanzo beans - 2 cans.

Feta cheese – 1/2 cup.

Preparation

Keep the feta cheese aside and mix the remaining ingredients in a small bowl. After about half hour top it with cheese.

Grapefruit, Raw Kale And Hazelnut Salad

Grapefruit is an ideal fruit for those who are trying to shed some pounds. This fruit contains lot of water and they are full of nutrients. Studies have proved that consuming this fruit on a regular basis can help us in losing weight faster.

Ingredients

Pink grapefruit – 2

Thinly sliced red onion – 1/2 onion

Lemon juice – 1/4 cup

Fat-free yogurt – 1/2 cup

Extra-virgin olive oil – 2 tbsp.

Kosher salt – 1/2 tbsp.

Black pepper – 1/4 tbsp.

thinly sliced lacinato kale – 8 ounces

Toasted and chopped hazelnuts – 1/3 cup

Preparation

Peel the grapefruit and squeeze few of the pieces to make 3 tbsp fresh juice. Take 2 slices of onion and mince them well. Mix it with the grapefruit juice and add yogurt, lemon juice, salt, oil and pepper. Stir all the ingredients to form a mixture.

Add the kale and then add rest of the grapefruit, onion and hazelnuts.

Avocado Whip

Avocado whip can be served as a dip or a spread. It is a healthy dish that can boost your metabolism and accelerate the fat-burning process.

Ingredients

Peeled avocados – 2.

Lime juice – 1/4 cup.

Tahini – 1 tbsp.

Chopped onion -1/4 cup.

Kosher salt -1/4 tbsp.

Fresh pepper – 1/4 tbsp.

Preparation

Keep aside 1 tablespoon of lemon juice. Mix everything in a food processor and process the mixture for 30 seconds. Now sprinkle the lime juice and refrigerate the mixture. While serving sprinkle some pepper.

Banana And Almond Butter

This is an easy dish and it is perfect for breakfast. Almond butter contains ingredients that reduce hunger. Apart from rare nutrients, almonds also contain monounsaturated fats.

Ingredients

Almond butter – 1 tbsp.

Toasted bread – 1 slice.

Sliced banana – 1

Preparation

Spread the almond butter evenly on the toast.

Arrange the banana slices on the toast.

All these recipes are quite interesting and innovative. They are not only delicious and different, but they are made of foods that promote fat burning and weight loss. Most of the recipes contain fruits and vegetables that promote metabolism. If you are on a weight-loss regimen, then try to follow these special diets. Replace your regular menu with these fat-burning and gluten-free recipes. They can definitely help you in cutting back several extra pounds.

www.ingramcontent.com/pod-product-compliance
Lightning Source LLC
Chambersburg PA
CBHW071303280526
45788CB00004B/1823